Off The Wall Contrarian Quotes For
People In Recovery

Off The Wall Contrarian Quotes For People In Recovery

Tuchy Palmieri

2007

Off The Wall Contrarian Quotes For People In Recovery

Dedication: This collection of quotes, adages, sayings, and points to ponder are a result of years of involvement and guidance from many people familiar with the 12-step program of Alcoholics Anonymous and offshoots such as Overeaters Anonymous. I want to thank the many people in my life who introduced me to recovery programs, especially Raymond Fitch, who suggested I go to A.A. and Al-Anon meetings.

To M. Scott Peck, who advised all attendees at one of his workshops to find an excuse to get into any 12-step program. To my dear friend John Moser, who labored over theses writings to insure their accuracy and applicability; to Dale Kesten, my friend who helped me so much to find answers. And to my wife, Susan Palmieri, who has supported me through thick and thin in my pursuit of self-discovery. And finally to our wonderful children; Kathleen, Phil, Amy, John, and Stephen.

This book is also dedicated to all the people in all recovery programs, especially to the sponsors, who carry the message.

In loving memory of my brother, Joe Palmieri

INTRODUCTION

PLEASE NOTE: THESE WRITINGS ARE NOT
APPROVED BY A.A. OR BY ANY OTHER
PROGRAM

The intention is that this collection of sayings, quotes, and
thoughts brings help to recovering people. From a simple
laugh to helpful insights, and in the spirit of taking what
works and leaving the rest, you are encouraged to do so.

QUOTATIONS ABOUT BOOKS AND READING

A good book on your shelf is a friend that turns its back on you and remains a friend.

-Author Unknown

Anyone who says they have only one life to live must not know how to read a book.

-Author Unknown

Let books be your dining table,
And you shall be full of delights
Let them be your mattress
And you shall sleep restful nights.

-Author Unknown

A book is like a garden carried in the pocket.

-Chinese proverb

A dirty book is rarely dusty.

-Author Unknown

BIG BOOK/ GOOD BOOK QUOTES

1) One must be careful that they do not get so hot that they melt their clay feet and lose their footing.

2) Be glad you are off the wall; it gives one freedom to move.

3) A slip is when you stop doing the same thing over and over and expecting the same result.

4) When you are in the rooms and not doing the steps you are only safe if you can walk on dangerous waters.

5) The alcoholic proved the proverb that watch out for your friends and love your enemies. Their friend alcohol became their enemy and their enemies became their friends.

FAST ON FEAR; FEAST ON FAITH.

BIG BOOK/GOOD BOOK QUOTES-CONTINUED

6) I never knew an insane person who did not know.

7) The progress of prayer—pray to, pray for, pray with.

8) We are told ask and you shall receive, so if you have not received you may not have asked enough.

9) How politicians see the 12 steps: the conservative sees God, the liberal has a higher power, the independent sees a universal force, and the green party sees love and tolerance.

10) You alone have no power; you and the group high power, God higher power, you and God the highest power for you.

One night a man had a dream. He dreamed he was walking along the beach with the Lord. Across the sky flashed scenes from his life. For each scene he noticed two sets of footprints in the sand: One belonged to him and the other to the Lord.

When the last scene of his life flashed before him, he looked back at the footprints in the sand. He noticed many times along the path of his life there was only one set of footprints. He also noticed that it happened at the very lowest and saddest times in his life.

This really bothered him and he questioned the Lord about it. Lord, You said that once I decided to follow You, You'd walk with me all the way. But I have noticed that during the most troublesome times in my life there is only one set of footprints. I don't understand why when I needed You most You would leave me. The Lord replied, "my precious, precious child, I love you and I would never leave you during your times of trial and suffering. When you see one set of footprints, it was then that I carried you."

-Author Unknown

BIG BOOK/GOOD BOOK QUOTES-CONTINUED

11) Contrarian promises: you will feel good about shameful acts, you will embrace your character defects, and you will know real insanity.

12) The disease of alcoholism is like the disease of cancer; if left unchecked they will take your life.

13) When you follow more than one path you are never sure which one is right.

14) It makes no difference who inspires you, friend or foe; it just matters that you are inspired.

15) The only time some people go through the doors of a church is to attend a 12-step meeting.

FAST ON SELF-PITY AND FEAST ON GRATITUDE.

BIG BOOK/GOOD BOOK QUOTES CONTINUED

16) Hazelden books — the apocrypha of the 12 steps.

17) Just because you think good does not mean you are a good thinker.

18) Strange, Bill and Dr. Bob did not recover by reading the big book.

19) Jesus did not read the Bible.

20) When you stop doing the steps you are actually taking a step backwards.

AA SLOGANS

It works…it really does! (Page 88, line 8 in the big book)

More will be revealed.

It's in the book.

When all else fails, follow directions.

Respect the anonymity of others.

Principles before personalities.

When we surrender to our higher power, the journey begins.

Fear stands for Frustration, Ego, Anxiety, and Resentment.

The 12 steps tell us how it works; the 12 traditions tell us why it works.

When man listens, God speaks; when man obeys, God works.

Your big book is your sponsor too.

BIG BOOK/GOOD BOOK QUOTES CONTINUED

21) It is strange but you actually slip when you stop rather than when you are taking steps.

22) It is the only place where you can slip when you stop.

23) The big book: one of the books that spreads the good news.

24) The real old-timers: the prophets of the big book.

25) The trinity of the 12 steps: spiritual, emotional, and physical.

FAST ON ISOLATION; FEAST ON FELLOWSHIP.

BIG BOOK/GOOD BOOK QUOTES CONTINUED

26) 12 steps: the other trinity.

27) The big book—the drinking man's bible.

28) At first it loosens the tongue, then it twists it, and finally it quiets the tongue.

29) With recovery you are either recovering or you are not.

30) Beware of the Pharisees of the program.

31) Christ—the original protestant.

As children bring their broken toys,
With tears for us to mend,
I brought my broken dreams to God,
Because He is my friend.
But then instead of leaving Him
In peace to work alone,
I hung around and tried to help,
With ways that were my own.
At last, I snatched them back again
And cried, "How can you be so slow?"
"My child," He said, "What could I do?
You never did let go."

-Author unknown

BIG BOOK/GOOD BOOK QUOTES CONTINUED

32) You must leave the convex and concave mirrors in your life for the true mirrors in the fellowship.

33) The problem may not be that you are out of your mind but rather in your mind.

34) A.A. proves that history repeats itself.

35) Question: Who did Bill and Dr. Bob follow?

36) It's the miracle of turning from wine to water.

FAST ON SELF-WILL; FEAST ON GOD'S WILL

BIG BOOK/GOOD BOOK CONTINUED

37) The food of the program will never harm you.

38) The fellowship—brotherly love healing hearts.

39) The medicine prescribed by the program brings you relief from your disease. It is not for everyone. Consult with your sponsor to see if the 12 steps are for you. The side effects are peace, joy, love, serenity, happiness, and a conscious contact with God. Do not take this medicine if you suffer from the inability to be honest or if you are unwilling to be willing.

40) The Bible proves that the message of the written word changes.

41) The A.A. big book is a program guide based upon principles similar to the biblical teachings.

42) The A.A. big book is a program based upon ancient and universal principles.

HUMILITY

Humility is the recognition of the allness of God
And the nothingness of self.

It is the lowly root that stiffens the great oak
Against storms of the centuries.

It is the father of confidence, the mother of joy,
The brother of courage, the sister of kindness.

It walks with wisdom,
Talks with truth,
And dwells with love.

True humility is not a garment, but a trait of character.

It never intrudes, often has to be discovered, it is never
boisterous nor self-assertive.

But if it is mistaken for weakness there is apt to be a rude
awakening, for the strength of humility lies in its impersonal
selflessness, a fundamental element of power.

It adds power to authority, credence to reason, and
reverence to spirituality.

THE BIG BOOK

1) The big book is like the good book in many ways...neither should be taken literally.

2) The problem with the big book comes when you don't take it literally.

3) The big book is actually on the small side, as far as books go.

4) For ME reading the big book is good; and reading it with the good book is better.

5) A dishonest mistake—a lie.

AA SLOGANS

Easy does it.

Live and let live.

One day at a time.

Let go and let God.

Expect miracles.

Keep coming back...it works if you work it.

Keep an open mind.

Pass it on.

90 meetings in 90 days...90/90.

Use the 24-hour plan.

Call your sponsor before, not after, you take the first drink.

Help is only a phone call away.

Keep coming back...kcb.

THE PROGRAM

1) It's where you discover you have not asked God enough.

2) It turns flaming idiots into balls of fire that go around lighting everyone's candle.

3) It's where people get religion.

4) For some people the program is their religion of choice.

5) One of the purposes of the program is to examine insanity.

HOW THE PROGRAM FEEDS US:

It satisfies our hunger for appreciation.

It satisfies our hunger for acceptance.

It satisfies our hunger for the wanted to be heard.

It satisfies our hunger for self-acceptance.

It satisfies our hunger for health.

THE PROGRAM-CONTINUED

6) Some call it magic.

7) The program is about changing your thinking from over thinking to rethinking.

8) Program instruments: a drum, a horn, and a fiddle.

9) Program utensils: a can opener, spatula, tongs, and a nutcracker.

10) A program that takes a person out of his mind and out of the world.

11) Program tools: a hammer, an air compressor, a drill, a broom, and a jackhammer.

1. You will receive a body.
You may like it or hate it, but it will be yours for the entire period this time around.

2. You will learn lessons.
You are enrolled in a full-time, informal school called "life." Each day in this school you will have the opportunity to learn lessons. You may like the lessons or think them irrelevant and stupid.

3. There are no mistakes, only lessons.
Growth is a process of trial and error, experimentation. The "failed" experiments are as much a part of the process as the experiment that "works."

4. A lesson is repeated until it is learned.
A lesson will be presented to you in various forms until you have learned it. Then you can go on to the next lesson.

-Author unknown

PONDERING THE STEPS

1) Some people do the steps by sidestepping.

2) Some people take such small steps that they never get their feet high enough to the ground.

3) Skipping steps is one of the surest ways to slip.

4) Even a normal person will slip if he tries to skip steps.

5) Going back one step can be a giant step forward.

6) If you turn around before you take a step, you will never go backwards.

1. Learning lessons does not end.
There is no part of life that does not contain its lessons. If you are alive, there are lessons to be learned.

2. "There" is no better than "here."
When your "there" has become a "here," you will simply obtain another "there" that, again, looks better than "here."

3. Others are merely mirrors of you.
You cannot love or hate something about another person unless it reflects to you something you love or hate about yourself.

4. What you make of your life is up to you.
You have all the tools and resources you need; what you do with them is up to you. The choice is yours.

5. The answers lie inside you.
The answers to life's questions lie inside you. All you need to do is look, listen, and trust.

-Author unknown

PONDERING THE STEPS-CONTINUED

7) Sidestepping is the way we get stuck.

8) When you find that you are stuck on a step, check to see if you are sidestepping.

9) Side-stepping does not move you forward.

10) If your steps are not built on the foundation of God, then you will eventually crumble.

11) For me the 12 steps are about uncovering your tracks and walking in the footsteps of God.

12) The steps go both ways.

Our Father, who art in Heaven

Hallowed be thy name.

Thy Kingdom come, Thy will be done,

On Earth as it is in Heaven.

Give us this day our daily bread and forgive us our trespasses

As we forgive those who trespass against us.

And lead us not into temptation

But deliver us from evil

For Thine is the Kingdom, the Power, and the Glory forever.

Amen.

PONDERING THE STEPS-CONTINUED

13) Members need the steps to pick them up and others need the steps to take them down.

14) Not doing the steps is like having a toothache and not doing anything about it. Sooner or later the ache will take you down, as will any disease.

15) Some people want the steps to do them.

16) Some people want the steps to take the action. (John Moser)

17) To take the recovery path you must take steps.

FAST ON RESENTMENT; FEAST ON FORGIVENESS.

PONDERING THE STEPS-CONTINUED

18) Desire earns you a seat in the rooms; taking the steps keeps placing you there.

19) You are finished once you finish with the steps.

20) Where the journey begins after the final step.

21) The least valid statement in the program: "I have finished the steps."

22) Some people are willing to go to any steps rather than go to all lengths.

23) Some people are willing to go to different steps rather than go to any length.

SIGNS OF A SPIRITUAL AWAKENING

1. An increased tendency to let things happen rather than make them happen.

2. Frequent attacks of smiling.

3. Feelings of being connected with others and nature.

4. Frequent overwhelming episodes of appreciation.

5. A tendency to think and act spontaneously rather than from fears based on past experience.

6. An unmistakable ability to enjoy each moment.

-Source unknown

GENERAL PONDERING

1) An honest lie—one you believe in.

2) Make sure the diamond in the rough is not just an ordinary piece of coal.

3) A piece of coal is but a diamond in the rough.

4) You really do not have to be one to know one.

5) A dishonest mistake—a lie.

6) Too many of us corrected our honest mistakes with dishonest ones.

7) I never knew an insane person who did not know.

MORE SIGNS OF A SPIRITUAL AWAKENING

1. A loss of ability to worry.

2. A loss of interest in conflict.

3. A loss of interest in interpreting the actions of others.

4. A loss of interest in judging others.

5. A loss of interest in judging self.

6. Gaining the ability to love without expecting anything in return.

-Source unknown

GENERAL PONDERING-CONTINUED

8) How strange; as you get stronger you pick up less, if at all.

9) Hitting your bottom is like depression—it is the first step towards feeling better.

10) Hitting your bottom is the first step towards getting better.

11) Bottoms up is one of the surest ways to hit your bottom.

12) A high bottom is not on one's body.

13) Asking a roach to deroach himself is like asking a tiger to remove his stripes.

14) A point to ponder—is accepting the things you cannot change an act of serenity, or an act of sanity?

15) Not being normal can be a very good thing.

"How would it be if just for today we thought less about contests and rivalries, profits and politics, winners and sinners and more about helping and giving, mending and blending, reaching out and pitching in? How would it be?"

-Anonymous

GENERAL PONDERING-CONTINUED

16) Do not ask if you are normal or not, but ask what side of normal you are.

17) The only difference between sanity and insanity is the time we are acting in each.

18) A question: If a sane person performed an insane act is he really insane? Conversely, if an insane person did a sane act, is he sane?

19) An insane act can make a sane person insane, and yet a sane act by an insane person does not make him sane.

20) If you ask enough people, all apples are bad.

21) I am sorry for those of us who are normal as they are not free.

22) It is possible to get good fruit from a bad tree.

23) Going to any length includes all length.

FAST ON SADNESS; FEAST ON HAPPINESS.

GENERAL PONDERING-CONTINUED

24) Not all mirrors reflect back at you.

25) The mirror you are using may not reflect back properly.

26) A big shot is not very big at all—about one-and-a-half ounces.

27) If you are going to shoot the messenger at least wait until the message has been delivered.

28) Disorganization is a key to success.

29) The signs on the road you travel depend upon the direction you are traveling.

30) Being grateful for being able to have your round peg in a square hole.

BE THANKFUL

Be thankful that you don't already have everything you desire.
If you did, what would there be to look forward to?

Be thankful when you don't know something.
For it gives you the opportunity to learn.

Be thankful for the difficult times.
During those times you grow.

Be thankful for your limitations.
Because they give you opportunities for improvements.

Be thankful for each new challenge.
Because it will build your strength and character.

Be thankful for your mistakes.
They will teach you valuable lessons.

Be thankful when you're tired and weary.

A life of rich fulfillment comes to those
Who are also thankful for the setbacks.

Find a way to be thankful for your troubles
And they can become your blessings.

GENERAL PONDERING-CONTINUED

31) What a sad world it would be if everything fit perfectly and worked perfectly.

32) The disease is like a cockroach; you can never eliminate it, you can only control it with a de-roaching process.

33) I hit my bottom in '87 and hit my top in '91.

34) I prefer being off the wall than being a still life on the wall.

35) If you are not off the wall then you are not moving and have a still life.

36) Does a fly on the wall really care what you are saying or are doing?

37) The messenger can change the meaning of the words without changing the words.

38) Do not try to change the messenger rather than changing the words.

FAST ON REGRET; FEAST ON APPRECIATION.

GENERAL PONDERING-CONTINUED

39) Changing the messenger does not change the message.

40) I know you know it all, but I'm not sure you know that all you know is not all there is to know.

41) It is a verbal book club that listens to the same stories over and over again.

42) It is a program of reciprocal promises.

43) The question is, do you see it as a spiritual program of recovery, or is it a program of spiritual recovery?

44) Sobriety allows one to begin their emotional and spiritual recovery.

45) Making a decision is a good start; acting on it is success.

Holding your head high, and being the best you know you can be when life seems to fall apart at your feet, facing each difficulty with the confidence that time will bring you better tomorrows, and never giving up,
...means confidence.

-Author unknown

GENERAL PONDERING-CONTINUED

46) Taking what is said out of the rooms is a sin against the program.

47) An attitude of gratitude increases your altitude and enables you to soar above the turbulence of life.

48) When an alcoholic is drinking he has fear and he gets frozen in his tracks; when the alcoholic gets sober he has the courage to stand on high ground.

49) When an alcoholic is drinking he has fear and he gets stiff in the gutter; when the alcoholic gets sober he has the courage to stand on high ground.

50) It is important to grasp the point that he knows he's not all there; then he is able to grasp the will of God.

51) Just because you are moving, that does not mean you are taking the steps.

52) An INACTIVE alcoholic—one who is active with the steps.

FAST ON CRITICISM; FEAST ON PRAISE.

GENERAL PONDERING-CONTINUED

53) Making a decision in step three is a good start; acting on it is success.

54) One who has accepted his calling.

55) To give is more powerful than to receive.

56) Bill Wilson—an example of the power of giving over receiving.

57) The critical step is when a person takes to making amends.

58) A fellowship of believers who trust in God and believe they received a gift in order to give it away.

59) Let us not forget the real intent of a boomerang is to give you a second chance.

60) Think less; do more.

1) Faith instead of despair.

2) Courage instead of fear.

3) Hope instead of desperation.

4) Peace of mind instead of confusion.

5) Real friendship instead of loneliness.

6) Self-respect instead of self-contempt.

7) Self-confidence instead of helplessness.

8) A clean conscience instead of a sense of guilt.

9) The respect of others instead of their pity and contempt.

10) A clean pattern of living instead of a hopeless existence.

11) The love and understanding of our families instead of their doubts and fears.

12) The freedom of a happy life; not the bondage of an alcoholic obsession.

THE 12 STEPS

1) Some people believe they can recover by sidestepping.

2) The 12 steps are straight and narrow; if you sidestep you will fall off the path.

3) Practicing the 12 steps is the best way to learn how to stay on the wagon.

4) There are two kinds of people in the 12-step program: those who step too, and those who step on others.

5) God is the railing in the 12-step program that you must hold onto for support as you do the steps.

6) Doing the steps requires you to pick up your feet.

7) Make sure the 12 steps you are taking are not taking you in circles.

STEP ONE satisfies our hunger for truth and awareness.

STEP TWO satisfies our hunger for hope.

STEP THREE satisfies our hunger for help.

STEP FOUR satisfies our hunger for inner cleansing.

STEP FIVE satisfies our hunger to disclose the undiscloseable.

STEP SIX satisfies our hunger for God's help.

THE 12 STEPS-CONTINUED

8) A 12-stepper knows his mind is wasted.

9) A person doing the 12 steps will tell you that the mind is not a terrible thing to waste.

10) The 12 steps is akin to a recycling station; garbage in, clean material out.

11) In the context of the 12-step literature, bigger is better.

12) The big book— the 12-step bible.

13) The 12-step program teaches you that you do not need variety to have spice in your life.

14) The 12 steps is a process in which you are softened so that you can be remolded by the hands of God.

STUFF THAT MAKES YOU FEEL GOOD

Think about each one for a while before going on to the next...

Falling in love.

Laughing so hard your face hurts.

A special glance.

Getting mail.

Taking a drive on a pretty road.

Hearing your favorite song on the radio.

Lying in bed listening to the rain outside.

Hot towels fresh out of the dryer.

Finding the sweater you want is on sale.

A chocolate milk shake. (Or vanilla) (Or strawberry).

A long-distance phone call.

A bubble bath.

THE 12 STEPS-CONTINUED

15) In the 12 steps we first listen to ourselves, then we listen to others, and finally we learn to listen to God.

16) Another 12-step definition of insanity: making changes over and over, expecting the results to stay the same.

17) Some people only need to take twelve steps on the pathway to God.

18) The 12-step program makes it ok to not be ok.

19) The 12 steps can be seen as the ultimate Protestant Movement.

20) The 12 steps are where you have insights about your insights.

21) Churches, synagogues, temples, and halls play a great role in the 12-step program. For some it's by going and others by not going.

22) A 12-stepper is a disciple of Bill and Doctor Bob.

MORE STUFF THAT MAKES YOU FEEL GOOD

Giggling.

A good conversation.

Finding $20 in your coat from last winter.

Running through sprinklers.

Laughing for no reason at all.

Friends.

Overhearing someone say something nice about you.

Watching the sunrise.

Your first kiss.

Making new friends or spending time with old ones.

Playing with a puppy.

Sweet dreams.

THE 12 STEPS-CONTINUED

23) A 12-stepper is an insane person who is no longer mad.

24) A 12-stepper is a reformed mad man.

25) On the recovery path there are 12 steps and three bridges—physical, emotional, and spiritual.

26) Pigeon—the unofficial bird of the 12 steps.

27) 12 steps—use universal laws to solve a specific problem.

28) Contrary to popular belief the 12 steps prove a closed mind leads to an opened heart.

29) A recovering 12-stepper—an anonymous missionary.

30) 12 steps is a treatment program that when done on a consistent basis prevents the disease from spreading.

LIFE ISN'T ABOUT FINDING
YOURSELF. LIFE IS ABOUT CREATING
YOURSELF.

MEETING ROOMS

1) In the rooms we find that insanity is changing something and expecting the same result.

2) It's strange—when you first come in you hear stories about good things.

3) It's where you learn to feel good about the bad.

4) In the rooms is where you learn to talk a good game.

5) In the rooms is where talk is not cheap.

6) In the rooms is where saying your piece brings you peace.

7) It's where people tell real-life stories about terrible things in such a way that it makes the people in the room happy.

8) It's where you can treat someone like dirt with love and tolerance.

MEETINGS SATISFY HUNGER FOR FELLOWSHIP, AND QUENCH OUR THIRST FOR FRIENDSHIP.

MEETING ROOMS-CONTINUED

9) It's where people go to hear stories about the good, the bad, and the ugly.

10) In the rooms is where you can hear yourself without speaking.

11) The way to get to a meeting room is to take the low road.

12) A place where despicable and shameful acts are applauded.

13) In the rooms is where the powerless become powerful.

14) In the rooms you learn that forgiveness is an act of self-love.

15) In the rooms you learn to tolerate intolerance.

16) In the rooms is where you are told true love stories.

WHAT KIND OF DAY SHALL I CHOOSE TODAY?

Today I can complain about my health,
Or I can celebrate being alive.

Today I can moan that it is raining,
Or be joyful at all that grows from the rain.

Today I can regret all I don't have,
Or rejoice in everything I do.

Today I can complain that I have to work,
Or celebrate having a job to go to.

Today I can resent the mess the kids make,
Or give thanks that I have a family.

Today I can whine about the housework,
Or celebrate having a home.

Today I can cry over those who don't care for me,
Or be happy loving and being loved by those who do.

I choose to have a good day!

MEETING ROOMS-CONTINUED

17) In the rooms is where you find that the most important meeting is with yourself.

18) Meetings are where you meet yourself.

19) Meetings—where wounded birds flock together.

20) If you listen in on a 12-step meeting you find that the meetings are a series of re-meetings.

21) If you met someone outside the rooms and every time they spoke to you they would start by saying, "hi" and giving their name, you would think they were insane.

22) What I like about the 12-step meetings is that you can never be late and never leave early.

23) Meetings—where the undecided decide.

24) Meetings—where you get the good news from the big book.

25) It's a place where you can come in high and leave even higher.

THE PROGRAM SATISFIES ONE'S HUNGER FOR:

Self-worth through service

Peace by doing the steps

Freedom by turning it over to God

Happiness by the fellowship and God connection

MEETING ROOMS-CONTINUED

26) It's a place where you come in low and leave high.

27) It is where you are taught to not listen, to stop thinking, and begin unlearning.

28) It is where I really learned not to listen.

29) It is where I really learned not to hear but to listen.

30) It is where I was taught not to think.

31) Meetings—a place to air your dirty laundry.

32) In the churches, synagogues, and meeting halls you hear the word of God. In the rooms you see the words of God.

33) You can find a meeting at the crossroads of heaven and hell.

SERENITY PRAYER

God grant me the serenity
To accept the things I cannot change,
Courage to change the things I can,
And the wisdom to know the difference.

Living one day at a time;
Enjoying one moment at a time;
Accepting hardship as the pathway to peace.

Taking, as He did, this sinful world
As it is, not as I would have it;

Trusting that He will make all things
Right if I surrender to His will;

That I may be reasonably happy
In this life,
And supremely happy with Him
Forever in the next.

-Reinhold Niebuhr

THE PROGRAM/FELLOWSHIP

1) When I came into the program I was in such bad shape I couldn't even fall off the wagon.

2) The program proves that being a bad example can be a good example.

3) The program teaches strange math—it's where you can exchange one 1/5 for another and make a whole.

4) In the program you fill the holes to become whole.

5) It's where you can treat someone like dirt with love and tolerance.

6) It's where the insane go to get sane.

THE PROGRAM SATISFIES ONE'S HUNGER FOR:

Human connection through the fellowship

Know serenity through action

Usefulness through sponsorship

Economic security through following God's will

Handling baffling situations by letting God help

THE PROGRAM/FELLOWSHIP-
CONTINUED

7) The program takes those who have risen above the crowd and brings them back to earth.

8) The people in the program took the low road to get to the high road.

9) Instead of rubbing elbows you learn to touch hearts.

10) The magic of the program is that you end up feeling good about your bad deeds.

11) The program takes you to the far side of insanity.

12) The program is like Disneyland—there is something for everyone to enjoy.

"When you come to the edge of all the light you know and are about to step off into the darkness of the unknown, faith is knowing one of two things will happen: There will be something solid to stand on or you will be taught to fly."

-Author Unknown

THE PROGRAM/FELLOWSHIP-CONTINUED

13) The program is like a zoo—you get to see real animals.

14) The program is about embracing your insanity to get sane.

15) If you are in the rooms year after year and are not doing the steps you are actually stepping on the program.

16) The program is nonresistance in action.

17) In the program you come in thinking you're sane. The program immediately starts off by convincing you that you are insane. Next they ask you to embrace your insanity, and finally you finish by being grateful for your insanity. Now that's insane.

18) Many people come into the rooms wanting to get a jump on it. The program tells them to take it easy.

ALTERNATE SERENITY PRAYER

God grant me the serenity to accept the people I cannot change directly,

The courage to change the person I can,

The wisdom to know that person is me,

And to leave the changes of others to God and them.

THE PROGRAM/FELLOWSHIP-CONTINUED

19) Some people in the program got there because they tried to captain two ships at the same time.

20) Many in the program say they are recovering Catholics. I say I am a recovering alcoholic and compulsive overeater who is Catholic.

21) The program—collective deroaching.

22) The program—collective debugging. (John Moser)

23) The program works much better if you do not ask what it can do for you, but rather ask what you can do for it.

GRATITUDE AND APPRECIATION

Any and all compliments can be handled by simply saying, "Why, thank you" (though it helps if you say it with a Southern accent).

Appreciation is a wonderful thing; it makes what is excellent in others belong to us as well. (Voltaire)

Be glad of life because it gives you the chance to love and to work and to play and to look at the stars. (Henry Van Dyke)

Be happy while you're living, for you're a long time dead. (Scottish proverb)

The best and most beautiful things in this world cannot be seen or even heard, but must be felt with the heart. (Helen Keller)

THE PROGRAM/FELLOWSHIP CONTINUED

24) The program asks you for commitments and upon keeping those, the program gives you what it promises.

25) A program of mutual commitment.

26) In the program you are not asked to try, but to work.

27) You learn in the program what works is work.

28) The only requirement to be a member of a 12-step program is a desire to stop. The only requirement for recovery is a willingness to go to any length.

MORE GRATITUDE AND APPRECIATION

Blessed are those who can give without remembering and take without forgetting.

The capacity of delight is the gift of paying attention. (Julia Cameron)

A cloudy day is no match for a sunny disposition. (William Arthur Ward)

Don't cry because it's over; smile because it happened.

Don't ever save anything for a special occasion. Being alive is the special occasion.

THE PROGRAM/FELLOWSHIP-CONTINUED

29) The program teaches you to own your problems so that your problems do not own you.

30) The program is actually about reprogramming.

31) A program result, because you are heard, you can then be quiet, and hear the word of God.

32) The medicine prescribed by the program brings you relief from your disease. It is not for everyone. Consult with your sponsor to see if the 12 steps are for you. Side effects are peace, joy, love, serenity, happiness, and a loving God.

33) The program takes you from know-it-all to one who knows that he does not know it all and is content with not knowing it all, and knowing who knows it all.

FRIENDSHIP

"The better part of one's life consists of his friendships."
-Abraham Lincoln

"A true friend is one who overlooks your failures and tolerates your success."
-Anonymous

"The road to a friend's house is never long."
-Danish proverb

"Books and friends should be few but good."

"A friend in need is a friend indeed."
-Latin proverb

THE PROGRAM/FELLOWSHIP-CONTINUED

34) A program of reciprocal promises.

35) Working the program halfway is akin to reaching middle ground—you may be out of immediate danger but if you do not move to high ground you will soon be wet.

36) A fellowship of believers who trust in God and that they will receive a gift in order to give it away.

37) Other program tools—a hammer, an air compressor, a drill, a broom, and a jackhammer.

38) The program is about changing your thinking from over-thinking to rethinking.

FRIENDSHIP

"Do not use a hatchet to remove a fly from your friend's forehead."
-Chinese proverb

"The death of a friend is equivalent to the loss of a limb."
-German proverb

"Life without a friend is like death without a witness."
-Spanish proverb

"The best mirror is an old friend."

THE PROGRAM/FELLOWSHIP-CONTINUED

39) Program instruments—a drum, a horn, and a fiddle.

40) A program that takes a person out of his mind and his world.

41) The program is like a magnet—it works on the law of attraction.

42) You commit to the program and the program commits to you.

43) A paradox of the program is that when you stop trying and start working, the program works.

44) Secret society where secrets are told and kept.

45) The program is about turning the tide.

IN THE WORDS OF GEORGE BERNARD SHAW, PARAPHRASED:

"This is the true joy in life —

Being used for a purpose, recognized by yourself as a mighty one.

Being a force of nature, instead of a feverish, selfish little clod of ailments and grievances, complaining that the world will not devote itself to making you happy.

I AM OF THE OPINION THAT MY RECOVERY BELONGS TO THE WHOLE COMMUNITY AND AS LONG AS I LIVE IT IS MY PRIVILEGE TO DO FOR IT WHATEVER I CAN."

RECOVERY

1) You are recovering when you reach the other side of insanity.

2) You are recovering when you near the side of sanity. (John Moser)

3) Recovery—a grateful alcoholic.

4) A recovering Catholic is one who uses the program to have love and tolerance with the church and uses the principles of the program in their religious affairs.

5) Believing that you have recovered is the start of your relapse.

6) It is the only recovery program in which you are not expected to fully recover.

"May there always be work for your hands to do, may your purse always hold a coin or two. May the sun always shine on your windowpane, may a rainbow be certain to follow each rain. May the hand of a friend always be near you, may God fill your heart with gladness to cheer you."

-Irish blessing

RECOVERY-CONTINUED

7) Recovery comes when you hear another voice.

8) Do you see it as a spiritual program of recovery or is it a program of spiritual recovery?

9) Sobriety allows one to begin their emotional and spiritual recovery.

10) Recovery is an attitude of gratitude with fortitude.

11) Recovery is action that believes in itself.

12) Recovery—what matters over the mind.

TO "LET GO" TAKES LOVE

To "let go" does not mean to stop caring,
It means I can't do it for someone else.

To "let go" is not to cut myself off, it is
The realization I can't control another.

To "let go" is not to enable, but to allow
learning from natural consequences.

To "let go" is to admit powerlessness, which
means the outcome is not in my hands.

To "let go" is not to care for, but to care about.
To "let go" is not to fix, but to be supportive.
To "let go" is not to judge, but to allow another
to be a human being.

To "let go" is to not regret the past,
but to grow and to live for the future.
To "let go" is to fear less and to love more.

-Source Unknown

STEP NUMBER ONE

No man is an island
No man is an island
No man is an island
No man is an island
No man is an island
No man is an island
No man is an island
No man is an island
No man is an island
No man is an island

I cannot do it alone
I cannot do it alone
I cannot do it alone
I cannot do it alone
I cannot do it alone
I cannot do it alone
I cannot do it alone
I cannot do it alone
I cannot do it alone
I cannot do it alone

FORGIVE US OUR DEBTS

Loose the cords of mistakes binding us,
As we release the strands we hold
Of others' guilt.

Forgive our hidden past, the secret shames
As we consistently forgive
What others hide.

Lighten our load of secret debts as
We relieve others of their
Need to repay.

Absorb our frustrated hopes and dreams,
As we embrace those of others
With emptiness.

Compost our inner, stolen fruit
As we forgive others the spoils of
Their trespassing.

Loose the cords of mistakes binding us,
As we release the strands we hold
Of others' guilt.

STEP NUMBER TWO

It can happen
It can happen
It can happen
It can happen
It can happen
It can happen
It can happen
It can happen
It can happen
It can happen
It can happen
It can happen
It can happen
It can happen
It can happen
It can happen

EMPTIED OF MYSELF

Sever me from myself that I may be grateful to you;
May I perish to myself that I may be safe in you;
May I die to myself that I may live in you;
May I wither to myself that I may blossom in you;
May I be emptied of myself that I may abound in you;
May I be nothing to myself that I may be all to you.

-Erasmus

STEP NUMBER THREE

1) A sobering thought

2) Making a promise to the program

3) Soul power

4) Perpetual power

5) Thou shall have one spirit, not many spirits before you.

6) Thou shall have one God and not many liquid spirits before you. (John Moser)

7) Thou shall have but one spirit within you.

8) I have given up the spirits for one spirit—the Holy Spirit.

KNOW MYSELF

I thank you Lord for knowing
Me better than I know myself,

And for letting me know myself
Better than others know me.

Make me, I ask you then, better
Than they suppose,

And forgive me for what they do not know.

-Abu Bakr

STEP NUMBER FOUR

1) Requires you to go backward to go forward.

2) Requires you to look backward in order to go forward. (John Moser)

3) Inventory is a spiritual balance sheet.

4) It is about uncovering your steps.

5) It is the crane that clears away life's wreckage and allows you to begin rebuilding.

IN THE WORDS OF GEORGE BERNARD SHAW, PARAPHRASED:

"I WANT TO BE THOROUGHLY USED UP WHEN I DIE.

For the harder I work the more I live.

I rejoice in life for its own sake.

Life is no longer the brief candle it was when I was addicted.

It's a sort of splendid torch, which I've got to hold up for the moment and I want to make it burn as brightly as possible before handing it on to future generations of recovery."

STEP NUMBER FOUR-CONTINUED

6) The untold story

7) Writing your wrongs

8) After you have gone down the yellow brick road you can take the road to recovery back home.

9) To take the recovery path you must take steps.

10) Clear away the wreckage of your past; in step 9 you salvage it.

11) A big shot is not very big—just about two ounces.

NO EASY ANSWERS

May God bless me with discomfort at easy answers,
Half truths, and superficial relationships,
So that I may live deep within my heart.

And may God bless me with tears for those
Who suffer from pain, rejection and starvation, and war,
So that I may reach out my hand to comfort them.

And to turn their pain into joy.

-Anonymous

STEP NUMBER FIVE

1) Go where you have not gone before.

2) Letting the cat out of the bag.

3) Spilling the beans on yourself.

DIFFICULTIES

It is not easy:
To apologize,
To being over,
To be unselfish,
To take advice,
To admit error,
To face sneers,
To be charitable,
To avoid mistakes,
To keep on trying,
To be considerate,
To endure success,
To profit by mistakes,
To forgive and forget,
To think and then act,
To keep out of the rut,
To make the best of little,
To subdue an unruly temper,
To maintain a high standard,
To shoulder a deserved blame,
To recognize a silver lining.
But it always pays!

STEP NUMBER SIX

Opened arms
Opened arms
Opened arms
Opened arms
Opened arms
Opened arms
Opened arms
Opened arms
Opened arms
Opened arms

THE PRAYER OF ST. FRANCIS

Lord, make me a channel of thy peace,
That where there is hatred, I may bring love;
That where there is wrong, I may bring the spirit of
forgiveness;
That where there is discord, I may bring harmony;
That where there is error, I may bring truth;
That where there is doubt, I may bring faith;
That where there is despair, I may bring hope;
That where there are shadows, I may bring light;
That where there is sadness, I may bring joy.

Lord, grant that I may seek rather to comfort than to be
comforted;
To understand, than to be understood;
To love, than to be loved.

For it is by self-forgetting that one finds.
It is by forgiving that one is forgiven.
It is by dying that one awakens to Eternal Life.

STEP NUMBER SEVEN

1) Validates the power of prayer.

2) On your knees.

3) Ask humbly; listen honestly.

4) I ask humbly and listen honestly; God's will becomes very clear.

5) Ask humbly; listen honestly and you will clearly see.

VOICE IN THE WINDS

O Great Spirit,
Whose voice I hear in the winds
And whose breath gives life
To all the world,
Hear me! I am small and weak.
I need your strength and wisdom.
Let me walk in beauty
And make my eyes
Ever behold the sunset.
Make my hands respect the things
You have made.
And my ears sharp to hear your voice.
Make me wise
So that I may understand
The things you have taught my people.
Let me learn the lessons
You have hidden in every leaf and rock.
I seek strength,
Not to be greater than my brother,
But to fight my greatest enemy—myself.
Make me always ready to come to you
With clean hands and straight eyes.
So when life fades, as the fading sunset,
My spirit may come to you without shame.

STEP NUMBER EIGHT

The "did-to" list
The "did-to" list
The "did-to" list
The "did-to" list
The "did-to" list
The "did-to" list
The "did-to" list
The "did-to" list
The "did-to" list
The "did-to" list

THE RIGHT ROAD

O Lord God,
I have no idea where I am going,
I do not see the road ahead of me,
I cannot know for certain where it will end.
Nor do I really know myself.
And the fact that I think I am following your will
Does not mean that I am actually doing so.
But I believe that the desire to please you
Does in fact please you.
And I hope I have that desire in all that I am doing.

...I will trust you always
Though I may seem to be lost
And in the shadow of death
I will not fear,
And you are ever with me,
And you will never leave me,
To make my journey alone.

STEP NUMBER NINE

1) It is important not to step on anyone.

2) Teaches you that telling the truth may not always be the right thing to do.

3) Telling the truth may not always be right. (John Moser)

4) He is a normal person in his own mind.

5) Desire earns you a seat in the rooms; taking the steps keeps placing you there.

6) Getting on your knees is encouraged to help you pray; getting up is encouraged to help you stay.

7) The steps actually work on you, but at first you must work them.

STEP NUMBER NINE

Satisfies our hunger for peace and forgiveness.

STEP NUMBER NINE-CONTINUED

8) Working the steps is like kneading dough; if you keep doing it you will eventually rise.

9) Where the journey begins after the final step.

10) The least valid statement in the program: I have finished the steps.

11) You are finished once you finish with the steps.

12) One of the goals of the program is to awaken the spirit and to put to bed the suffering.

13) A spiritual awakening occurs when you stop shooting the messenger and receive the message.

14) If you are going to shoot the messenger at least wait until the message has been delivered.

15) Traditions 8: we are a bunch of amateurs.

I RISE TODAY

I rise today through
God's strength to pilot me,
God's eye to look before me,
God's ear to hear me,
God's word to speak for me,
God's hand to guard me,
God's way to lie before me,
God's shield to protect me,
God's hosts to save me
From the snares of the devil,
From everyone who desires me ill
From afar or near, alone or in a crowd.

-Saint Patrick

STEP NUMBER TEN

1) Is six steps in one

2) Made up of smaller steps

3) Is a dance you do everyday

4) Is the Texas two-step

5) Is the exception to the rule

6) One step at a time except for step ten

STEP NUMBER TEN

Satisfies our daily hunger.

STEP NUMBER TEN-CONTINUED

7) If you find yourself too busy on the tenth step to get to steps 11 and 12 you may need to make more amends.

8) An act of daily reflection, confession, and amends

9) An admission that even with all the step work you will find that you will continue to do wrong on occasion.

10) A recognition of the fact that in spite of making a decision to turn our will and our lives over to the care of God, and of having done the steps, you will continue to make mistakes.

11) The whetstone that keeps you sharp

12) When 4 and 5 make 10

13) Perpetual confession

TEACH ME TO SING

Giver of Life, Creator of all that is lovely
Teach me to sing the words of your song.

I want to feel the music of living
And not fear the sad songs
Composed of both laughter and tears.

Teach me to dance to the sounds of your world
And your people
I want to move in rhythm with your plan.

Help me to follow your leading
To risk even falling
To rise and keep trying
Because you are leading the dance.

-Author unknown

STEP NUMBER ELEVEN

1) We see the wisdom when it's said through prayer and meditation.

2) Requires that you do more than pray.

3) Pray for the willingness to meditate before step 11.

4) Wisdom can be seen more effectively when we look at the numbers separately, 1 is for prayer and 1 for meditation; both are needed.

5) The contrarian eleventh step—silent prayer speaking meditation.

6) Unconscious contact with God—when good things happen to you and you say, "what happened?"

7) Message morphs when you have many messengers.

FOR TODAY

O God:

Give me strength to live another day;
Let me not turn coward before its difficulties;
Let me not lose faith in other people;
Keep me sweet and sound of heart,
In spite of ingratitude, treachery, or meanness;
Preserve me from minding little stings or giving them;
Help me to keep my heart clean,
And so to live so honestly and fearlessly
That no outward failure can take away the joy of conscious integrity;
Open wide the eyes of my soul that I may see good in all things;
Grant me this day some new vision of thy truth;
Inspire me with the spirit of joy and gladness;
And make me the cup of strength to suffering souls;

In the name of the strong Deliverer,
Our only Lord and Savior, Jesus Christ.

STEP NUMBER TWELVE

Spiritual awakening occurs after the mind is quieted and the ego is put to sleep.

Spiritual awakening occurs after the mind is quieted and the ego is put to sleep.

Spiritual awakening occurs after the mind is quieted and the ego is put to sleep.

Spiritual awakening occurs after the mind is quieted and the ego is put to sleep.

Spiritual awakening occurs after the mind is quieted and the ego is put to sleep.

Spiritual awakening occurs after the mind is quieted and the ego is put to sleep.

PERSISTENCE

Nothing in the world can take the place of persistence.

Talent will not; nothing is more common than unsuccessful men with talent.

Genius will not; unrewarded genius is almost a proverb.

Education will not; the world is full of educated derelicts.

Persistence and determination alone are omnipotent.

-Calvin Coolidge

PROGRAM PSALMS

"Amazing Grace"

"Nearer My God to Thee"

"We Call on Him"

"I Walk in the Garden Alone"

"Standing on the Promises"

"My Prayer"

"All I Have to Do Is Dream"

"How Great Thou Art"

"It's All in His Hands"

"Peace in the Valley"

"You Are My Sunshine"

PEACE

It does not mean to be in a place where there is no noise, trouble, or hard work. It means to be in the midst of those things and still be calm in your heart.

-Unknown

PROGRAM PROVERBS

1) Serenity, letting go, and helping God.

2) Skipping steps keeps you off balance.

3) Enlightenment springs from the manure of the mind.

4) Take a tip from the big book and revise yourself.

5) Honesty is about uncovering your tracks.

6) Will power and want power give way to higher power.

7) Put your disease at ease, and when it is at ease it's no longer a disease.

8) You cannot do the steps sitting on your high horse.

Service to others is the crowning glory of one's being. The gift one is given to be of service to one who is suffering is a gift that never wears out, always stays fresh, can be taken in small bites, feeds others, and nurtures oneself. May I always look to be of service to my fellow human being who still suffers.

PROGRAM PROVERBS-CONTINUED

9) Exchange the shot and a beer for love and tolerance.

10) Tolerance is when the tolerant tolerate the intolerant until the intolerant become tolerant.

11) Getting high brings you to the bottom.

12) Insanity—choosing your lower power.

13) When you receive, don't ask.

14) Most apples are bad.

15) A great example can be good or bad.

16) What is the cost of a free ticket?

17) It is possible to get good fruit from a bad tree.

ANONYMITY SATISFIES HUNGER
FOR SECURITY AND QUENCHES THE
THIRST FOR PRIVACY.

PROGRAM PROVERBS-CONTINUED

18) A soft answer turneth away wrath: but grievous words stir up anger.

19) The tongue of the wise useth knowledge aright: but the mouth of fools poureth out foolishness.

20) The eyes of the LORD are in every place, beholding the evil and the good.

21) A wholesome tongue is a tree of life: but perverseness therein is a breach in the spirit.

22) A fool despiseth his father's instruction: but he that regardeth reproof is prudent.

23) In the house of the righteous is much treasure: but in the revenues of the wicked is trouble.

LITERATURE SATISFIES HUNGER FOR GUIDANCE AND QUENCHES THE THIRST FOR INFORMATION.

PROGRAM PROVERBS-CONTINUED

24) The lips of the wise disperse knowledge: but the heart of the foolish doeth not so.

25) The sacrifice of the wicked is an abomination to the LORD: but the prayer of the upright is his delight.

26) The way of the wicked is an abomination unto the LORD: but he loveth him that followeth after righteousness.

27) Correction is grievous unto him that forsaketh the way: and he that hateth reproof shall die.

28) Hell and destruction are before the LORD: how much more then the hearts of the children of men?

29) A scorner loveth not one that reproveth him: neither will he go unto the wise.

30) A merry heart maketh a cheerful countenance: but by sorrow of the heart the spirit is broken.

WRITING SATISFIES HUNGER FOR CLARITY, AND QUENCHES THE THIRST FOR RECORDING.

PROGRAM PROVERBS-CONTINUED

31) You cannot hit a home run sitting in the bleachers.

32) Highest power: when God's will and your will are perfectly aligned.

33) Work works.

34) The baptism of your rebirth

35) HALT: happy, aligned, loving, and tolerant.

36) GO: god only.

37) A sponsor: the minister of the word.

FAST ON INSECURITY; FEAST ON SECURITY.

PROGRAM PROVERBS-CONTINUED

38) A prayer a day helps keep the doctor away.

39) It takes a heart to open a heart.

40) The liquor of love makes you drunk on life.

41) Recovery starts when the arguing stops.

42) Recovery: when you lose.

43) Platinum became more precious than gold because of its usefulness.

44) The road even less traveled.

45) Serenity: finding a round hole for your round peg.

46) Spiritual minds think alike.

47) Think less; do more.

Biggest Handicap- Fear

Most Beautiful Day- Today

Easiest Thing to Do- Give Up

Biggest Error- To Quit

Biggest Fault- Self-Centeredness

Best Gift- Faith

Greatest Need- Good Sense

Worst Sentiment- Jealousy

Best Present- A Pardon

Best Christian- Mary

Most Beautiful Thing in the World- Love

TRADITIONS

Tradition 1: United we stand, divided we fall.

Tradition 2: When two or more are gathered in my name.

Tradition 3: Unconditional acceptance.

Tradition 4: Guided by God only.

Tradition 5: Minister.

Tradition 6: To each his own.

FAST ON FEAR AND KNOW THAT
YOU CAN FEAST ON COURAGE.

TRADITIONS-CONTINUED

Tradition 7: A bunch of amateurs.

Tradition 8: Disorganization is the key to success.

Tradition 9: I hear nothing, I say nothing, and I see nothing.

Tradition 10: Behind closed doors.

Tradition 11: A closed-door session.

Tradition 12: A secret society helping a select few.

MIRACLES ARE EVERYWHERE

Miracles are not only
Ecstatic visions or holy
Interventions
Visited upon the chosen few.

Every moment we are alive
Is full of reasons to sing
Out in joyful gratitude.

Every breath we are given
Is a reminder that
The glory of life is at hand.

In the people we love,
In the beauty of nature,
In the golden sun
That rises each morning-
Miracles are everywhere.

M IRACLES

M Mary Martha Melissa Megan Marsha Melinda Matilda Maureen

I Irene Isabelle Ida Ilene Ingrid Iris Irma Ivonna Ivanka Ivory Ivy

R Rachael Rose Robin Rhoda Rita Rochelle Ronnie Rosa Rosalyn Ruth

A Ann Alice Amy Alisa Annette Alicia Ava Alvira Alyson Amanda

C Carol Carla Cindy Cathy Christine Caroline Carmella Carey Candy

L Linda Lisa Louise Lorie Lucia Lee Liz Laura Lola Lindsey Lea

E Ellen Elizabeth Evyone Evett Eileen Eve Eleanor Ethel Edythe

S Sally Susan Sara Sophia Sabrina Sandy Samantha Sandra

THIRD STEP PRAYER

God,

I offer myself to Thee
To build with me and to do with me as Thou wilt.

Relieve me of the bondage of self, that I may better do Thy
will.

Take away my difficulties, that victory over them may bear
witness
To those I would help of Thy Power, Thy love and Thy way
of life.

May I do Thy will always!

PRAYER AND MEDITATION

1) When praying remember to stop and meditate so that you may hear the answer.

2) God told us to pray and meditate in order that we can ask and receive.

3) Ask through prayer and receive through meditation.

4) Often we ask to get and seldom we ask to give.

5) Careful you are not so busy praying for answers that you do not hear the response.

6) Praying is good; praying with meditation is better.

MIRACLES

M Michael Martin Murray Mickey Mark Malcolm Manuel Morris

I Ines Ingram Irving Irvin Isaac Isaiah Issa Ishmael Israel Igore Ivan

R Richard Robert Rolland Ryan Russell Randy Ricky Randall Rusty

A Albert Alan Art Amos Alex Aladdin Alexander Alfred Alec

C Carl Charles Clark Chris Carmon Chuck Craig Carlo Christian

L Louie Lincoln Larry Lonny Lenny Lawrence Lionel Lucky Lou

E Edward Edwin Evert Evan Ellis Evin Edgar Eddy

S Samuel Sammy Scott Stuart Stanley Sandy Sean Sal Shawn

PRAYER AND MEDITATION-CONTINUED

7) Powerful prayer is praying for the ones you love and the ones you do not.

8) If you start your day on your knees and end your day on your knees that is very good; by adding the act of sitting quietly for God's word it becomes better.

9) Meditation proves that sitting on your rear can be the most effective move you can make.

10) Prayer and belief go hand in hand; prayer without belief is but a wish.

11) How strange; at first you admit your powerlessness, then you pray for power to your higher power.

TWELFTH STEP PRAYER

Dear God,

My spiritual awakening continues to unfold.

The help I have received I shall pass on and give to others,
Both in and out of the Fellowship.

For this opportunity I am grateful.

I pray most humbly to continue walking
Day by day on the road of spiritual progress.

I pray for the inner strength and wisdom to practice

The principles of this way of life in all I do and say.

I need You, my friends, and the program every hour of
every day.

This is a better way to live.

THE TWELVE STEPS IN TWELVE MINUTES

Doing the twelve steps in twelve minutes:

"Dear Lord, I have made many mistakes. I'm tired of doing it wrong; I need your help, and I will follow You. I have hurt people along the way, especially you and I. I know that I have bad ways of being and stand ready for your miracle of grace. As I recount those I have hurt, I commit to you that from this day forward I will be vigilant about my actions and behavior; when I am wrong, I will confess to those I have wronged that day and to you. My prayer to You is to help me on my path, and to sit quietly so that my conscious contact with you expands."

LOVE

Love is a friendship that has caught fire. It is quiet understanding, mutual confidence, sharing and forgiving. It is a loyalty through good and bad. It settles for less than perfection and makes allowances for human weaknesses.

Love is content with the present, it hopes for the future and it doesn't brood over the past. It's the day-in and day-out chronicle of irritations, problems, compromises, small disappointments, big victories and working toward common goals.

If you have love in your life, it can make up for a great many things you lack. If you don't have it, no matter what else there is, it's not enough.

LOVE

1) Love and tolerance are the twin railings for the 12-stepper to hold on to.

2) Love: Tolerating the intolerant, until the intolerant become tolerant.

3) Love is when the unlovable are loved through their un-lovability to lovability.

4) Tough love is not really tough.

5) Tough love is when you do not let love get in the way of doing what is best for someone.

6) Acceptance—one part love, one part tolerance.

FAST ON UPSET; FEAST ON SERENITY.

LOVE-CONTINUED

7) If you have tolerance of someone they experience tolerance; if you add love to tolerance they experience acceptance.

8) Add love to tolerance and you get acceptance.

9) Love and tolerate others as you love and tolerate yourself.

10) The program proves that love alone is not enough. You can love someone and not accept them; you can tolerate someone and not accept them, but you cannot love and tolerate someone and not accept them.

11) Having love and tolerance of oneself brings true peace.

12) Acceptance is when love meets tolerance.

THE THINGS THAT COUNT

Count your garden by the flowers,
Never by the leaves that fall.

Count your days by garden hours,
Don't remember clouds at all.

Count your nights by stars, not shadows.

Count your years with smiles, not tears.

Count your blessings, not your troubles.

Count your age by friends, not by years.

GOD

1) Commitment—making God's will superior to how you think or feel.

2) Peace comes when you align your will with God's.

3) If you start slipping, check to make sure you are still holding God's hand.

4) God grant me the serenity to know that I cannot change other people, the courage to change the person I can and to have the wisdom to know that that person is I.

5) Hearing God through ordinary people.

6) The right has God; the left has a higher party, and the independent have love and tolerance.

FAST ON DOUBT; FEAST ON BELIEF.

GOD-CONTINUED

7) You go from no power to high power to higher power to highest power.

8) You alone have no power; you and the group high power; God higher power; you and God the highest power for you.

9) God does not care what house you choose, as long as you choose a house that honors Him and respects others.

10) The God of your understanding does not change; just your understanding of Him.

11) The way you are asked to clean up your act is to first act as if, then act as God would.

12) Do you really want to find God's will?

STEP SIX SATISFIES OUR HUNGER FOR GOD'S HELP.

GOD-CONTINUED

13) It's a battle of wills—my will, their will, our will, God's will. You may win a battle or two but the only way to win the war is to side with God.

14) The one will that cannot be changed is God's will.

15) One will that you will get in trouble with when you challenge it is God's will.

16) Happy, joyous, and free; happy because of one's disease, joyous in spite of an incurable disease, and free because of not being normal.

17) My will, I will, their will, our will, your will.

18) WWGD? What would God do?

WHAT IS MEDITATION?

Meditation is the activity of calling to mind, and thinking over, and dwelling on, and applying to oneself, the various things that one knows about the works and ways and purpose and promises of God.

It is an activity of holy thought, consciously performed in the presence of God, under the eye of God, by the help of God as a means of communication with God. Its purpose is to clear one's mental and spiritual vision of God, and to let His truth make its full and proper impact on one's mind and heart.

It is a matter of talking to oneself about God and oneself; it is, indeed, often a matter of arguing with oneself, reasoning oneself out of moods and doubts and unbelief into a clear apprehension of God's power and grace.

GOD-CONTINUED

19) GOD: grace of divinity.

20) Serenity prayer for Contrarians: God grant me the serenity to accept that I may not change, the courage to keep working to change, and the wisdom to continue changing.

21) Guru: GOD and you.

22) Guru: GOD and your sponsor.

23) God grant me the serenity to know that I'm a round peg and would not fit into a square hole, and that I need to find a round hole or be square.

24) God's gratitude list—when you write down God's will for you in all aspects of your life.

25) Just as ignorance of the law is no excuse, not knowing God's will is unwillingness.

26) When your will is willing then you will know God's will.

27) God's home in your heart.

STEP SEVEN SATISFIES OUR
HUNGER TO LET GO AND LET GOD'S
FORGIVENESS COME.

GOD-CONTINUED

28) Quieting the mind allows you to hear the word of God.

29) It is far better to know God's will and tell Him you are not yet ready than to keep asking Him for His will and later saying, "I don't know."

30) If the kingdom of heaven is within, then God's home is in your heart.

31) Peace comes when you align your will with God's.

32) From the manure of the mind, when fed by God, becomes the fertilizer that helps one grow into a peach of a man.

33) If your steps are not built on the foundation of God, then they will eventually crumble.

34) For me the 12 steps is about uncovering your tracks and walking in the footsteps of God.

35) If you walk in the footsteps of GOD long enough people will begin to see you as one who walks on water.

36) Do not forget you are gathered in His name.

A PRAYER FOR BLESSED ACCEPTANCE

Dear God, in this moment I hold your acceptance.

You love me completely, just as I am.
You see my great potential within,
And you nurture my tender heart of compassion.

In this moment, I let your acceptance be my own.

I accept others as the children of God.

I hold high their inner greatness,
Always seeking to serve the highest and best within all
people.

And so it is.

HIGHER POWER

1) You learn to replace will power with higher power.

2) The right has God, the left has a higher power, and the independent have love and tolerance.

3) You go from no power to high power to higher power to highest power.

4) My will, I will, their will, our will, and your will.

GRATITUDE IS THE HEART'S MEMORY

Gratitude unlocks the fullness of life. It turns what we have into enough, and more. It turns denial into acceptance, chaos into order, confusion into clarity. It turns problems into gifts, failures into success, the unexpected into perfect timing, and mistakes into important events. Gratitude makes sense of our past, brings peace for today and creates a vision for tomorrow.

SERVICE

1) The more determined you are to give it away the more it comes back to you.

2) Service is your gift back to God; your continued recovery is his way of thanking you.

3) Reaching out extends your hand; reaching in extends your heart.

4) To extend the hand requires you to reach out; to extend the heart requires you to reach in.

BELIEVE

Believe in your questions, no matter how trifling.
They are the gateway to knowledge, wisdom and enlightenment.

Believe in your gifts, no matter how small; they are God's providence to your world,
To enrich it, to enable it, to bring it love.

Believe in your past, no matter how painful.
It is a unique book of history; Gospel Revelation of God's mercy and faithfulness.

Believe in your yearnings, no matter how subtle.
They are energy, urging you forward in your quest for God.

Believe in your sinlessness, no matter painted fingers.
They are only passing vestiges of fears,
Reminding you to forgive, to remain rooted in Love's reality.

PROMISES

We are going to know a new freedom and a new happiness.

1) The end result of the steps is enlightened insanity.

2) What amazes many people is that a recovering person is happy about being not okay.

3) Speaking reveals your insanity, and upon speaking you become silent.

4) The bottom line of A.A. is that it transfers the angry, sad, and confused alcoholic into a grateful one.

5) I am sorry for those of us who are normal as they are not free.

6) Are you restrained by the shackles of normalcy?

BELIEVE

Believe in your vision no matter the climb.
It is a mountain peak, calling you to experience God.

Believe in your ideas, no matter the doubts.
They are seeds, seeking nourishment, sunshine, life-giving water.

Believe in your neighbor, no matter the risk,
Each one is sent from God to walk with you.

Believe in your God, no matter the mist.
God is strong and trustworthy and cares for you.

ALL:

May the God who creates,
The God who redeems and
The God who makes us all holy,
Bless us and remain with us
Forever and ever. Amen.

PROMISES-CONTINUED

7) A miracle: only after people learn that they will not totally recover that they become happy, joyous, and free.

8) Happy, joyous, and free—happy because of one's disease, joyous in spite of an incurable disease, and free because of not being normal.

9) Physical recovery starts you on the road to happiness; emotional recovery makes it joyous, and spiritual recovery sets you free.

10) The steps actually work on you, but at first you must work them.

11) One of the goals of the program is to awaken the spirit and to put to bed the suffering.

I AM OKAY

I WILL READ EVERY DAY UNTIL THIS THINKING BECOMES MY THINKING.

1. I feel warm towards ME because I am a unique, one-of-a-kind person.

2. I am in charge of my life.

3. My first responsibility is to learn to love myself more and more.

4. I make my own decisions, take credit for the good ones and accept the consequences of the others.

5. I am not my actions; I am the one who acts.

6. It's nice to have other people's love and approval, but even without it, I can love and accept MYSELF.

7. It is not what happens to me that determines whether I feel good or bad, but my attitude towards those things that does.

8. I do not have to prove my worth or excellence. I need only express myself honestly and effectively.

THE ABOVE ARE GOALS. IF I THINK RIGHT, I WILL FEEL RIGHT!

WE WILL NOT REGRET THE PAST NOR WISH TO SHUT THE DOOR ON IT

1) Part of the program is about being a bad example.

2) It's strange that talking to someone about the worst things you have done helps them.

3) Character defect shows up under the microscope of the steps.

4) Sometimes I am a bad example of someone being good and other times I'm a good example of someone being bad.

5) Real physical recovery requires you to go beyond stopping.

6) Real physical recovery requires you to stop drinking and start exercising. (John Moser)

7) The good the bad and the ugly.

SPIRITUAL NEEDS:

Love
Hope
Faith
Wisdom
Knowledge
Peace
Trust
Principle of unity
Prayer
Worship
Meditation
Study

WE WILL COMPREHEND THE WORD "SERENITY" AND WE WILL KNOW PEACE

1) Every time you do a step, you make a step towards recovery.

2) It is where your blacklist is replaced with your gratitude list.

3) Recovery starts when the arguing stops.

4) Quieting the mind allows you to hear the word of God.

5) Be like a duck and take to water rather than drinking like a fish.

6) If the kingdom of heaven is within, then God's home is in your heart.

7) Once you let go you are free to bounce off the walls.

8) In the program is where you are encouraged to get out of your head and into your heart.

THE TEN STEPS

1) Moving out of Denial into AWARENESS.
2) Moving out of Shock into FEELING.
3) Moving out of Hopelessness into CONFIDENCE.
4) Moving out of Fear into SAFETY.
5) Moving out of Anger into FORGIVENESS.
6) Moving out of Guilt into SELF-FORGIVENESS.
7) Moving out of Shame into SELF-APPRECIATION.

Having moved past the more "negative" states, one can then complete the more "positive" ones.

8) GRATITUDE and APPRECIATION.
9) LOVE.
10) FAREWELL and RELEASE.

NO MATTER HOW FAR DOWN THE SCALE WE HAVE GONE, WE WILL SEE HOW OUR EXPERIENCE CAN BENEFIT OTHERS

1) The newcomer asks God to cure his problem; the old-timer thanks God for his problem.

2) In the twelve steps you learn that no one is 100% honest 100% of the time, but rather we have degrees of honesty.

3) A good story about something bad is better than a bad story about something good.

4) You learn to have good thoughts about something bad.

5) 12-step meetings—where you get to meet yourself.

6) The steps are the medications that arrest the disease.

7) You slip back into your disease when you fail to take your medication.

8) An enabler—one who loves someone to death.

9) In the rooms you meet a group of storytellers who know hundreds of stories and yet tell only one.

TWELVE WAYS TO BE MISERABLE

1. Wait for others to make you happy.

2. Blame everyone else for your unhappiness.

3. Use "if only" whenever you can regarding time, money, or friends.

4. Compare what you have with what others have.

5. Always be serious.

6. Take responsibility for everything all the time.

7. Try to please everybody all the time (never say "no").

8. Help others but don't let anyone help you.

9. Consider your own wants unimportant.

10. If anyone compliments you, discount it.

11. If anyone says anything, exaggerate it.

12. Always stay calm and cool.

THAT FEELINGS OF USELESSNESS AND SELF-PITY WILL DISAPPEAR

1) It turns flaming idiots into balls of fire that go around lighting everyone's candle.

2) Stop trying; start working.

3) Being out of your mind is actually a good thing...it is far better than being in your mind.

4) Heal the heart and you heal the mind.

TECHNIQUES FOR THINKING

1) Keep life simple.

2) Practice being satisfied.

3) Beware of indecision.

4) Practice cheerfulness.

5) Learn to like people.

6) Live and Let Live.

7) Use adversity.

8) Don't take yourself so seriously.

9) Have a sense of humor.

10) Practice objectivity.

11) Tolerate your own mistakes.

12) Forgive yourself.

WE WILL LOSE INTEREST IN SELFISH THINGS AND GAIN INTEREST IN OUR FELLOWS

1) Real humility requires some to forgive themselves for the thought that they were better than others.

2) Growing by the inspiration of others does not require you to accept the actions of others that inspire you.

3) Being inspired by those you honor and respect is good; being inspired by those you do not honor and respect is better.

4) It makes no difference who inspires you, friend or foe; it just matters that you are inspired.

5) Tolerance without love is just tolerance. Tolerance with love is acceptance.

6) When you tolerate someone without love, they experience tolerance; when you tolerate someone with love they experience acceptance.

I AM OKAY

I WILL READ EVERY DAY UNTIL THIS THINKING BECOMES MY THINKING.

1. I am free of animosity or resentment.

2. I am a success to the degree that I feel warm and loving towards ME.

3. I am kind and gentle with ME.

4. I live one day at a time, doing first things first.

5. I am patient because I have the rest of my life to grow.

6. Every experience of my life contributes to my personal growth.

7. No one in the world is one bit more or less important than I.

8. My mistakes or failures just prove that I am human.

THE ABOVE ARE GOALS. IF I THINK RIGHT, I WILL FEEL RIGHT!

WE WILL LOSE INTEREST-CONTINUED

7) A beginner finds that when he puts his drink down, his cup runneth over.

8) Before you strive to win the battle make sure it's the one you want to win.

9) In the program you find hearts healing hearts.

10) In the fellowship you discover it takes a heart to heal a heart.

11) The fellowship in action—hearts healing hearts.

12) He is a normal person in his own mind.

13) Hatred and resentment are the weeds in the garden of your mind while love and tolerance are the plants. Honesty and willingness are the fertilizers for your garden.

THE FIVE HINDRANCES TO GROWTH

1. Sense desire...future oriented.

2. Hatred; anger, ill will, annoyance, irritation.

3. Sloth/torpor/laziness...let me go to sleep.

4. Restlessness...jumping from one thing to the next.

5. Doubt (perhaps most difficult of all) doubt in oneself or what one has chosen to do..."I can't do it;" "why do I want to?"

SELF-SEEKING WILL SLIP AWAY

1) Spirituality requires some of us to give up the spirits.

2) 12-step meetings: where you get to meet yourself.

There is a power in our thoughts. We create our own surroundings by the thoughts we think. Physically, this may take a period of time, but spiritually it is instantaneous. If we understood the power of our thoughts, we would guard them more closely. If we understood the awesome power of our words, we would prefer silence to almost anything negative. In our thoughts and words we create our own weaknesses and our own strengths. Our limitations and joys begin in our hearts. We can always replace negative with positive.

Because our thoughts can affect this eternal energy, they are the source of creation. All creation begins in the mind. It must be thought first.

OUR WHOLE ATTITUDE AND OUTLOOK UPON LIFE WILL CHANGE

1) You are bribed with unbelievable promises that at first you do not believe.

2) Definition of insanity—doing the same thing over and over, knowing you will get the same result and praying that it would be different.

3) Resentment is cancer of the mind. If you do not kill it, it will kill you.

4) A 12-stepper is a person who sees that life sucks and does something about it.

5) Old-timer—one who HALTED (happy, aligned, loving, tolerant, enlightened, and dependable).

6) The successful old-timer—a beginner with years under his belt.

EMOTIONAL-PSYCHOLOGICAL NEEDS:

Affection
Understanding
Encouragement
Attention
Compliments
Compassion
Self-esteem
Fellowship
Be consulted
Respect
Acceptance
Friends
Responsibility
Fulfillment
Meaningful work
Privacy
Appreciation
Communication
Quiet

OUR WHOLE ATTITUDE-CONTINUED

7) Some people take steps; others do steps.

8) Bringing the little train that thought it could to life.

9) To the newcomer: after you have gone down the yellow brick road, you can take the road to recovery back home.

10) Working the steps is like kneading dough; if you keep doing it you will eventually rise.

11) The good news is that you can actually put a round peg in a square hole.

12) Life is not broken, nor needs to be fixed.

Our deepest fear is not that we are inadequate,
Our deepest fear is that we are powerful
Beyond measure.

It is our light, not our darkness, that most
Frightens us. We ask
Who am I to be brilliant,
Gorgeous, talented, fabulous?

Actually, who are you not to be?
You are a child of God.

Your playing small doesn't serve the world.
There's nothing enlightened about shrinking
So that other people
Won't feel insecure around you.

We are all meant to shine, as children do.

We were born to make manifest
The glory of God that is within us.

It's not just in some of us;
It's in everyone.

As we let our own light shine,
We give other people permission to do the same;

As we're liberated from our own fear,
Our presence automatically liberates others.

FEAR OF PEOPLE AND OF ECONOMIC INSECURITY WILL LEAVE US

1) The genuine baptism under fire.

2) Love and tolerate others as you love and tolerate yourself.

3) The program proves that love alone is not enough. You can love someone and not accept them; you can tolerate someone and not accept them, but you cannot love and tolerate someone and not accept them.

4) The 12-step program is where you are urged to be out of your mind.

5) Getting on your knees is encouraged to help you pray; getting up is encouraged to help you stay.

6) The fellowship: brotherly love healing hearts.

7) Do not be a turkey and be killed to make people happy.

8) Spiritual minds think alike.

9) Be like a babe and go listen to stories.

I am your constant companion. I am your greatest helper or heaviest burden. I will push you onward or drag you down to failure. I am completely at your command. Half the things you do you might just as well turn over to me, and I will be able to do them quickly, correctly.

I am easily managed—you must merely be firm with me. Show me exactly how you want something done, and after a few lessons I will do it automatically. I am the servant of all great people; and alas, of all failures as well. Those who are failures, I have made failures.

I am not a machine, though I work with all the precision of a machine plus the intelligence of a human being. You may run me for a profit or turn me for ruin—it makes no difference to me.

Take me, train me, be firm with me, and I will place the world at your feet. Be easy with me and I will destroy you.

Who am I?

I am habit.

-Anonymous

WE WILL INTUITIVELY KNOW HOW TO HANDLE SITUATIONS THAT USED TO BAFFLE US

1) The real winner focuses on the war and not the battle.

2) The program clears the dead trees in the forest so that you can see the trees that are trying to grow.

3) Let go of your thinking to find your right mind.

4) A beginner can get confused and try to take 12 steps instead of doing the 12 steps.

5) The mind is a good servant but a poor master.

6) Mastermind: making your mind your servant.

7) When your head is in the clouds it is hard to see the ground.

8) When your head is in the clouds you cannot see the path and you will get lost.

9) A miracle is an acknowledgement that an unexpected and good event occurred.

LETTER FROM A FRIEND

I just had to write to tell you how much I love you. Yesterday I saw you walking with your friends. I hoped that soon you'd want Me to walk along with you, too. So I painted you a sunset and whispered a cool breeze to refresh you. I waited—you never called—I just kept on loving you.

As I watched you fall asleep last night, I wanted to touch you. I spilled moonlight onto your face—trickling down your cheeks as so many tears. You didn't think of me; I wanted so much to comfort you.

I love you, oh, if you'd only listen. The wind whispers My love. I shout it to you in the thunder and compose love songs for you. I warm you with My sunshine and perfume the air with nature's sweet scent. My love for you is deeper than any ocean and greater than any need. If you'd only realize how I care.

My Dad sends His love. I want you to meet Him—He cares so. So, please, call on me soon. No matter how long it takes, I'll wait, because I love you!

Your friend,
Jesus

WE WILL SUDDENLY REALIZE THAT GOD IS DOING FOR US WHAT WE COULD NOT DO FOR OURSELVES

1) The weaker you are the more you pick up; and the stronger you are the less you pick up.

2) Where the spiritual meets the physical and gets emotional.

3) Where the emotional meets the physical and gets spiritual.

4) The Old Testament, the Sermon on the Mount, how a man thinketh, and the greatest thing in the world—LOVE.

5) The new testament of the twelve steps—the big book.

6) The twelve traditions are the commandments of the program.

7) It is where you can see miracles—the ignorant become wise; the unhealthy become healthy; and the blind can see.

8) We are all born saints; a few of us remain that way.

PHYSICAL NEEDS:

Food
Shelter
Water
Health
Rest
Elimination
Light
Sex

WE WILL SUDDENLY REALIZE-CONTINUED

9) Miracles happen for you when you believe.

10) The road to recovery requires you to cross the rivers of belief and willingness.

11) A spiritual awakening occurs when you stop shooting the messenger and receive the message.

12) It is far better to know God's will and tell Him you are not yet ready than to keep asking Him for His will and later saying, "I don't know."

13) If the kingdom of heaven is within, then God's home is in your heart.

14) The program teaches you to be a good soldier by following the commander.

15) The program takes you from know-it-all to one who knows that he does not know it all and is content with not knowing it all.

16) A philosophy in which one comes to the belief that he cannot live a good and decent life alone and that others can help him if he reaches out.

What I do today is important because I am exchanging one day of my life for it.

Every morning you are handed 24 golden hours. They are one of the few things in this world that you get free of charge. If you had all the money in the world, you couldn't buy an extra hour. What will you do with the priceless treasure? Remember, you must use it, as it is given only once. Once wasted you cannot get it back.

SPONSOR/SPONSORSHIP

1) Changing sponsors at will is good as long as you do not use your will to change the message.

2) The reason for a sponsor is to avoid the phenomenon of the passing of messages. When more than one messenger is used to carry the message it gets distorted.

3) A sponsor is like a nutcracker. He wants to break open the shell without cracking the nut.

4) It is a verbal book club that listens to the same stories over and over again.

5) It is a program of reciprocal promises.

6) The question is, do you see it as a spiritual program of recovery, or is it a program of spiritual recovery?

SPONSORSHIP SATISFIES HUNGER
FOR RECIPROCATION AND
QUENCHES THE THIRST FOR
HELPING OTHERS.

SPONSOR/SPONSORSHIP-CONTINUED

7) Sobriety allows one to begin their emotional and spiritual recovery.

8) Making a decision is a good start; acting on it is success.

9) Taking what is said out of the rooms is a sin against the program.

10) An attitude of gratitude increases your altitude and enables you to soar above the turbulence of life.

11) When an alcoholic is drinking he has fear and he gets frozen in his tracks; when the alcoholic gets sober he has the courage to stand on high ground.

12) When an alcoholic is drinking he has fear and he gets stiff in the gutter; when the alcoholic gets sober he has the courage to stand on high ground.

SPONSOR

1. One who assumes responsibility for another person or a group during a period of instruction, apprenticeship, or probation.

Sponsor—someone who supports or champions something

Supporter, patron

Benefactor, helper—a person who helps people or institutions

Backer, angel—invests in a theatrical production

Godfather—someone having a relation analogous to that of a male sponsor to his godchild

Godparent—a person who sponsors someone (the godchild) at baptism

Guarantor, warranter, warrantor, surety—one who provides a warrant or guarantee

Patroness, patronne—a woman who is a patron or the wife of a patron

Pillar of strength, tower of strength—a person who can be relied on to give support and comfort

SPONSOR/SPONSORSHIP-CONTINUED

13) It is important to grasp the point that he knows he's not all there; then he is able to grasp the will of God.

14) Just because you are moving, it does not mean you are taking the steps.

15) An INACTIVE alcoholic: one who is active with the steps.

16) Making a decision in step three is a good start; acting on it is success.

17) One who has accepted his calling.

18) To give is more powerful than to receive.

The 12-step programs have delivered to millions and millions of people who could not help themselves, and who could not be helped by conventional means. It is alternative medicine for the mind and spirit. It has been said that the twelve steps are America's 20th-century spiritual contribution to the world. I personally was told to find an excuse to get into a twelve-step program and am very glad I did.

SPONSOR/SPONSORSHIP-CONTINUED

19) Bill Wilson: an example of the power of giving over receiving.

20) The critical step is when a person takes to making amends.

21) A fellowship of believers who trust in God and believe they received a gift in order to give it away.

22) Let us not forget the real intent of a boomerang is to give you a second chance.

23) Think less; do more.